Snack Smart

LOW-CALORIE OPTIONS TO HELP YOU ACHIEVE YOUR WEIGHT LOSS GOALS

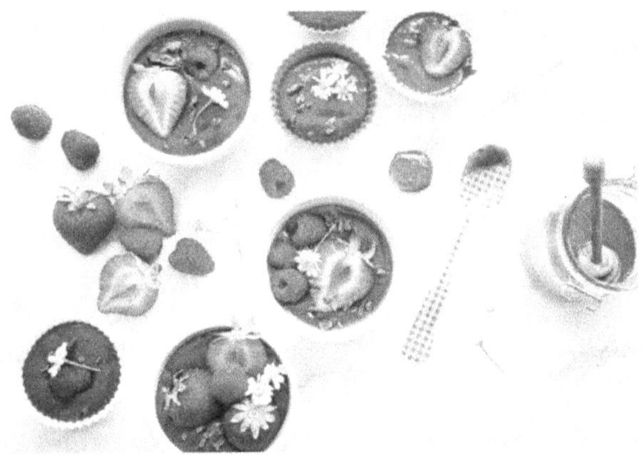

In this comprehensive guide to healthy snacking, you'll discover a wealth of delicious and satisfying low-calorie options that will keep you feeling full and energized throughout the day. Whether you're trying to lose weight or simply looking for nutritious snacks to fuel your busy lifestyle, "Snack Smart" provides a wealth of practical advice and mouth-watering recipes that will help you achieve your goals. With easy-to-follow tips and strategies for making smarter food choices, this book is the ultimate resource for anyone who wants to enjoy guilt-free snacking without sacrificing flavor or satisfaction.

"Snack Smart" is the ultimate guide to low-calorie snacking for weight loss. Written by a nutritionist, this book is packed with healthy and delicious snack ideas that will help you stay full and satisfied without derailing your diet.

Inside, you'll find a variety of snack options that are easy to prepare, portable, and perfect for any time of day. From crunchy veggies and protein-packed snacks to satisfying smoothies and guilt-free desserts, this book has something for everyone.

But "Snack Smart" is more than just a recipe book. It also includes helpful tips and tricks for making smarter snack choices, such as how to read nutrition labels, portion control, and healthy snacking on-the-go.

Whether you're just starting your weight loss journey or looking for new ideas to keep things fresh, "Snack Smart" is the ultimate resource for healthy snacking. With this book in hand, you'll be able to snack your way to your weight loss goals in no time!

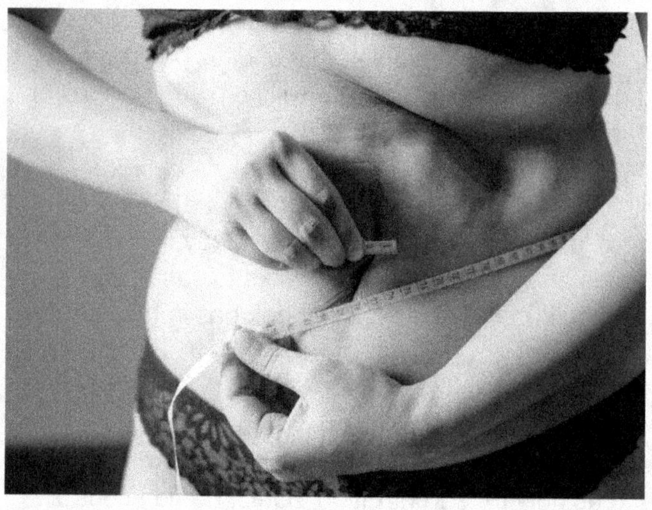

I. Introduction:

When it comes to losing weight, many people believe that snacking is a habit that should be avoided at all costs. However, the truth is that snacking can actually be a helpful tool in achieving your weight loss goals - as long as you do it smartly. Snacks can help keep hunger at bay between meals, preventing overeating and ensuring that you stick to your calorie budget for the day.

One of the keys to successful snacking for weight loss is choosing low-calorie options that provide important nutrients without packing on the pounds. In this guide, we'll explore the benefits of snacking on low-calorie options and provide you with plenty of delicious and satisfying snack ideas to help you reach your weight loss goals.

So why are low-calorie snacks so important? For starters, they allow you to indulge in the pleasure of snacking without consuming excess calories that can sabotage your weight loss efforts. Low-calorie snacks are also often high in fiber and protein, which can help keep you feeling full for longer and prevent overeating later in the day. Additionally, snacking on nutrient-dense, low-calorie options can provide your body with the vitamins and minerals it needs to stay healthy and energized.

In the following pages, we'll delve into the benefits of snacking smartly, and provide you with practical tips and tasty low-calorie snack ideas that will keep your taste buds happy while helping you achieve your weight loss goals. So grab a glass of water and let's get started!

II. Understanding Nutrition Labels

Explanation of the Key Information on Nutrition Labels:

Nutrition labels can provide important information about the nutritional content of packaged foods. By understanding the key information on these labels, you can make informed decisions about the foods you eat and work towards achieving your health and fitness goals.

One of the most important pieces of information on a nutrition label is the serving size. This tells you how much of the product is considered a single serving and is important to note because all of the other information on the label is based on this serving size. For example, if the serving size is half a cup of cereal, and you eat a full cup, you'll need to double all of the other numbers on the label in order to get an accurate understanding of the nutritional content of what you've eaten.

Another key piece of information on a nutrition label is the calorie count. This tells you how many calories are contained in a single serving of the product. For individuals who are trying to lose weight, paying attention to calorie counts can be an important part of managing their daily intake.

The nutrition label also provides information on the amount of fat, saturated fat, and trans fat in a product. Fat is an important macronutrient, but it's important to pay attention to the type and amount of fat you're consuming. Saturated and trans fats are generally considered less healthy than unsaturated fats, and should be consumed in moderation.

The nutrition label also provides information on the amount of carbohydrates, fiber, sugar, and protein in a product. It's important to note that not all carbohydrates are created equal - complex carbohydrates, such as those found in whole grains, are generally considered healthier than simple carbohydrates, which are often found in processed foods.

Finally, the nutrition label provides information on the vitamins and minerals that are contained in a product. This can be helpful for individuals who are trying to ensure that they're getting enough of certain nutrients in their diet.

Overall, paying attention to nutrition labels can be an important part of maintaining a healthy and balanced diet. By understanding the information on these labels, individuals can make informed decisions about the foods they eat, and work towards achieving their health and fitness goals

Tips for Reading and Interpreting Nutrition Labels:

a. Start with the serving size: As mentioned earlier, the serving size is an important piece of information on a nutrition label, as it sets the foundation for understanding the rest of the nutritional content. Be sure to pay attention to how many servings are in the package as well, as sometimes a single package can contain multiple servings.

b. Look for total calories: Knowing the total calories in a serving can help you determine whether the food fits into your daily calorie needs. Keep in mind that the calorie count on the label is based on one serving size, and you may need to adjust for the amount you actually eat.

c. Check for saturated and trans fats: Saturated and trans fats are generally considered less healthy than unsaturated fats, so it's important to limit your intake of these. Look for products that contain little or no saturated or trans fats, and try to choose healthier fats like those found in nuts, seeds, and fatty fish.

d. Look for fiber: High-fiber foods can help you feel fuller for longer and may also help with digestion. Try to choose products that contain at least 3 grams of fiber per serving.

e. Watch out for added sugars: Many packaged foods contain added sugars, which can contribute to weight gain and other health issues. Look for products that contain little or no added sugars, and be aware that sugar can appear on the label under many different names (such as sucrose, fructose, and corn syrup).

Common Pitfalls to Avoid When Reading Nutrition Labels:

a. Assuming the serving size is what you actually eat: As mentioned earlier, it's important to be aware of the serving size listed on the label and adjust the nutritional information accordingly.

b. Focusing solely on calories: While calories are an important piece of information, it's also important to pay attention to other nutrients like fat, fiber, and sugar.

c. Overlooking hidden sugars and fats: Some products may appear healthy but actually contain added sugars or fats. Be sure to read the entire label, including the ingredients list, to get a complete picture of what's in the food.

d. Relying solely on the front of the package: Many packaged foods feature claims like "low fat" or "low calorie" on the front of the package, but these claims can be misleading. Always check the full nutrition label to get the full picture.

By following these tips and avoiding common pitfalls, you can make informed decisions about the foods you eat and work towards achieving your health and fitness goals.

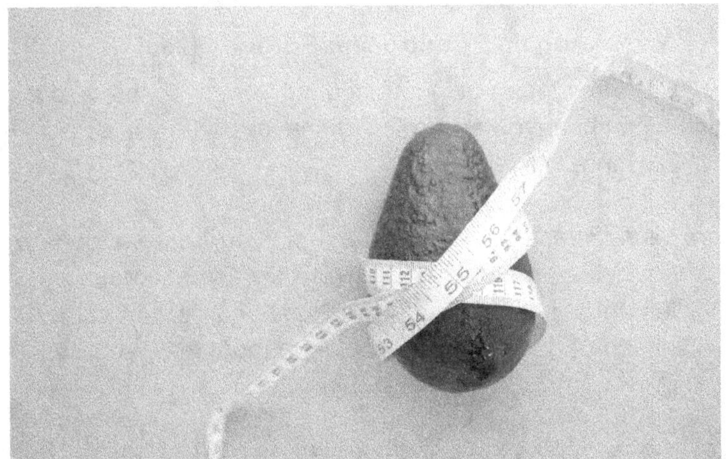

III. Portion Control

Explanation of the Importance of Portion Control:
Portion control is an important aspect of maintaining a healthy diet and managing your weight. When you eat more than your body needs, you consume excess calories that can lead to weight gain over time. By practicing portion control, you can ensure that you're eating the right amount of food to meet your nutritional needs without overindulging.

Tips for Measuring and Controlling Portion Sizes:

a. Use measuring tools: Using measuring cups, spoons, and a food scale can help you accurately measure portion sizes and avoid overeating.

b. Learn visual cues: Visual cues can help you estimate portion sizes when measuring tools aren't available. For example, a serving of meat should be roughly the size of a deck of cards, while a serving of rice or pasta should be about the size of a tennis ball.

c. Practice mindful eating: Paying attention to your food and eating slowly can help you feel full on less food, reducing the likelihood of overeating.

d. Use smaller plates and bowls: Using smaller plates and bowls can help you eat smaller portions without feeling deprived.

Strategies for Practicing Portion Control in Different Settings:

a. At home: Preparing and portioning meals and snacks in advance can help you avoid overeating. Store leftovers in single-serving containers for easy reheating later.

b. At work: Bring healthy snacks and meals from home to avoid the temptation of vending machines and fast food options. Use portioned containers to avoid overeating.

c. While traveling: Research healthy restaurant options in advance and order smaller portions or ask for a to-go box to save half for later. Pack healthy snacks for the journey to avoid overindulging in convenience store snacks.

By implementing these tips and strategies, you can take control of your portion sizes and maintain a healthy diet.

IV. Snack Ideas

A Wide Range of Low-Calorie Snack Ideas, Organized by Category:

a. Veggies:

Carrots, celery, and bell peppers with hummus
Cucumber slices with low-fat cottage cheese
Cherry tomatoes with a drizzle of balsamic vinegar
Sliced cucumbers with Greek yogurt dip
b. Fruits:

Apple slices with a tablespoon of almond butter
Berries with low-fat Greek yogurt
A small banana with a tablespoon of peanut butter
Grapefruit segments with a sprinkle of cinnamon
c. Protein-Packed Snacks:

Hard-boiled eggs
Edamame
Roasted chickpeas
Sliced turkey or chicken breast
d. Smoothies:

Spinach and banana smoothie with almond milk
Strawberry and kiwi smoothie with low-fat Greek yogurt
Pineapple and coconut milk smoothie with a scoop of vanilla protein powder
Blueberry and almond milk smoothie with chia seeds
e. Desserts:

Greek yogurt with a drizzle of honey and sliced almonds
Frozen grapes
Chocolate-covered strawberries (dip strawberries in melted dark chocolate and freeze)
Banana "ice cream" (blend a frozen banana until smooth and creamy)
By choosing low-calorie snacks that are rich in nutrients, you can satisfy your hunger and avoid overeating. These snack ideas are easy to prepare and can be enjoyed at home, work, or on the go.

2. Each snack idea includes nutritional information, preparation instructions, and tips for customization

here are some snack ideas with nutritional information, preparation instructions, and tips for customization:

a. Veggies:

1. Carrot sticks with hummus

- Nutritional Information: 1 medium carrot (61g) has 25 calories and 6g of carbs. 2 tablespoons of hummus (30g) has 70 calories and 5g of carbs.
- Preparation Instructions: Wash and peel the carrot, then cut it into sticks. Serve with hummus.
- Tips for Customization: Add some sliced cucumbers or cherry tomatoes for extra crunch and flavor.
1. Bell pepper slices with guacamole

- Nutritional Information: 1 medium red bell pepper (164g) has 40 calories and 9g of carbs. 2 tablespoons of guacamole (30g) has 50 calories and 2g of carbs.
- Preparation Instructions: Wash the bell pepper, remove the stem and seeds, then cut it into slices. Serve with guacamole.
- Tips for Customization: Try using different colors of bell peppers for a visually appealing snack or sprinkle some chili flakes on top for a spicy kick.

b. Fruits:

1. Banana and almond butter

- Nutritional Information: 1 medium banana (118g) has 105 calories and 27g of carbs. 1 tablespoon of almond butter (16g) has 100 calories and 3g of carbs.
- Preparation Instructions: Peel the banana and slice it into coins. Serve with almond butter.
- Tips for Customization: Top with some crushed almonds or sliced strawberries for some extra texture and flavor.

1. Apple and string cheese

- Nutritional Information: 1 medium apple (182g) has 95 calories and 25g of carbs. 1 piece of string cheese (28g) has 80 calories and 0g of carbs.
- Preparation Instructions: Wash and slice the apple, then serve with string cheese.
- Tips for Customization: Try using different types of apples for a variety of flavors or sprinkle some cinnamon on top for a cozy fall snack.

c. Protein-Packed Snacks:

1. Hard-boiled egg and cucumber slices

- Nutritional Information: 1 large hard-boiled egg (50g) has 70 calories and 0g of carbs. 1/2 cup of sliced cucumber (52g) has 8 calories and 2g of carbs.
- Preparation Instructions: Slice the hard-boiled egg and cucumber, then serve together.
- Tips for Customization: Add some smoked salmon or avocado for some extra healthy fats and flavor.

2. Turkey and cheese roll-ups

- Nutritional Information: 1 slice of deli turkey (28g) has 25 calories and 1g of carbs. 1 slice of cheddar cheese (21g) has 85 calories and 0g of carbs.
- Preparation Instructions: Lay the turkey slice on a plate and place the cheese on top, then roll it up and slice into bite-sized pieces.
- Tips for Customization: Use different types of cheese or try adding some sliced bell peppers or spinach for some extra nutrients.

d. Smoothies:

1. Kiwi and strawberry smoothie with Greek yogurt

- Nutritional Information: 1 medium kiwi (70g) has 35 calories and 8g of carbs. 1 cup of sliced strawberries (150g) has 50 calories and 12g of carbs. 1/2 cup of low-fat Greek yogurt (113g) has 60 calories and 4g of carbs.
- Preparation Instructions: Blend the kiwi, strawberries, and Greek yogurt until smooth.

- Tips for Customization: Add some spinach or kale for extra nutrients or use almond milk instead of yogurt for a dairy-free option.

2. Chocolate peanut butter banana smoothie

- Nutritional Information: 1 medium banana (118g) has 105 calories and 27g of carbs. 1 tablespoon of peanut butter (16g) has 95 calories and 3g of carbs. 1 cup of unsweetened almond milk (240g) has 40 calories and 2g of carbs. 1 tablespoon of unsweetened cocoa powder (5g) has 10 calories and 2g of carbs.
- Preparation Instructions: Blend the banana, peanut butter, almond milk, and cocoa powder until smooth.
- Tips for Customization: Try using different types of nut butter or add some protein powder for an extra boost of protein.

e. Desserts:

1. Frozen grapes and dark chocolate

- Nutritional Information: 1 cup of frozen grapes (92g) has 62 calories and 16g of carbs. 1 ounce of dark chocolate (28g) has 155 calories and 14g of carbs.
- Preparation Instructions: Wash the grapes and freeze for at least 2 hours. Melt the dark chocolate in a microwave or on the stove, then dip the grapes in the chocolate and let cool.
- Tips for Customization: Use different types of fruit or try sprinkling some chopped nuts on top for some extra crunch.

2. Greek yogurt and berry parfait

- Nutritional Information: 1/2 cup of low-fat Greek yogurt (113g) has 60 calories and 4g of carbs. 1/2 cup of mixed berries (75g) has 30 calories and 7g of carbs. 2 tablespoons of granola (10g) has 40 calories and 7g of carbs.
- Preparation Instructions: Layer the Greek yogurt, mixed berries, and granola in a glass or bowl.
- Tips for Customization: Use different types of fruit or try adding some honey or cinnamon for some extra sweetness and flavor.

These snack ideas are just a starting point - feel free to mix and match ingredients or add your own twist to suit your preferences and dietary needs. Remember to always check the nutrition label and portion sizes to ensure you are staying within your calorie and nutritional goals.

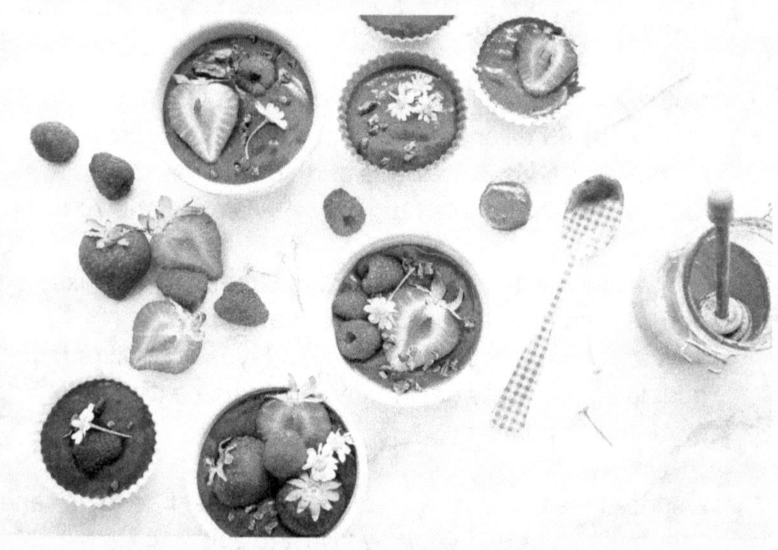

V. Conclusion:

1. Recap of Key Takeaways:

In this book, we've covered the importance of snacking for weight loss, how to read and interpret nutrition labels, the benefits of portion control, and a wide range of low-calorie snack ideas. Here are some key takeaways to keep in mind:

- Snacking can be an important part of a healthy weight loss plan, as long as you choose the right snacks and control your portion sizes.
- When reading nutrition labels, pay attention to the serving size, calories, and amounts of fat, sugar, and sodium.
- Portion control is essential for staying within your calorie and nutritional goals, and there are many strategies you can use to measure and control your portions.
- Low-calorie snacks can be delicious and satisfying, and there are many options to choose from in every food group.

2. Final Words of Advice for Incorporating Smart Snacking into a Healthy Lifestyle:

Incorporating smart snacking into a healthy lifestyle is all about balance and mindfulness. Here are some final tips to help you make the most of your snacks:

- Plan ahead and prepare your snacks in advance to avoid reaching for unhealthy options when you're hungry.
- Choose snacks that are nutrient-dense and high in protein and fiber to help you stay fuller for longer.
- Don't forget to enjoy your snacks mindfully - savor the flavors and textures, and pay attention to your body's hunger and fullness signals.

- And most importantly, be kind to yourself - healthy snacking is just one part of a healthy lifestyle, so remember to focus on progress, not perfection.

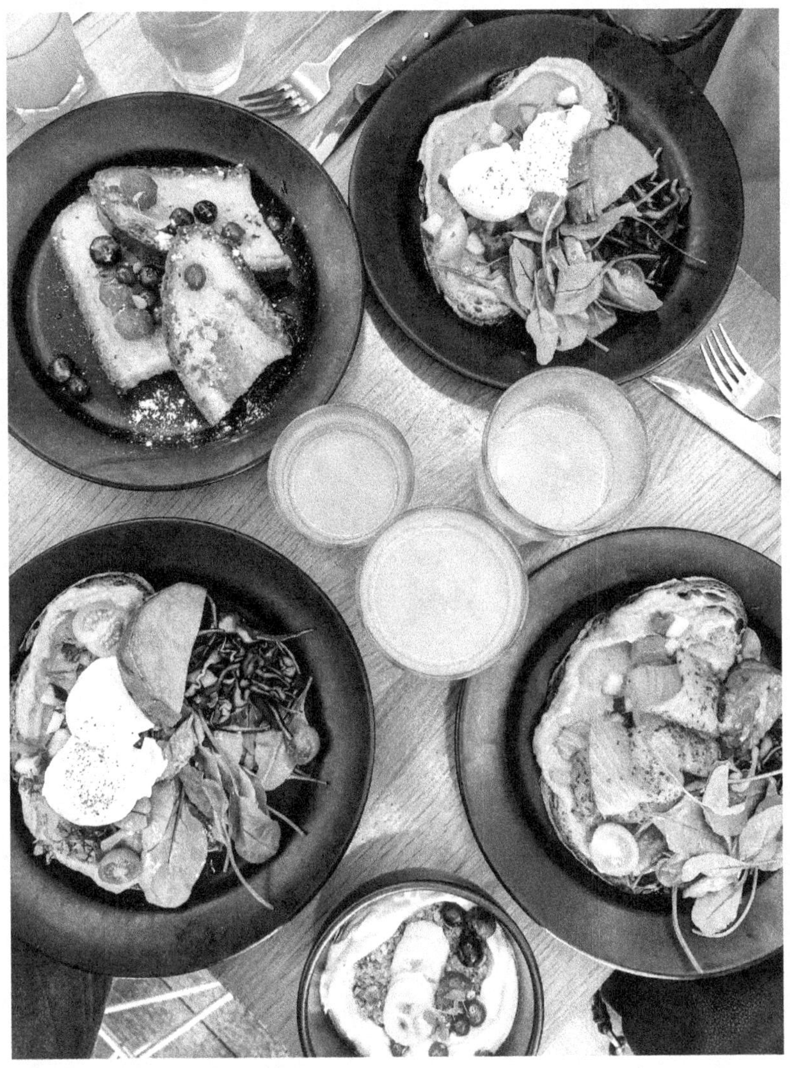

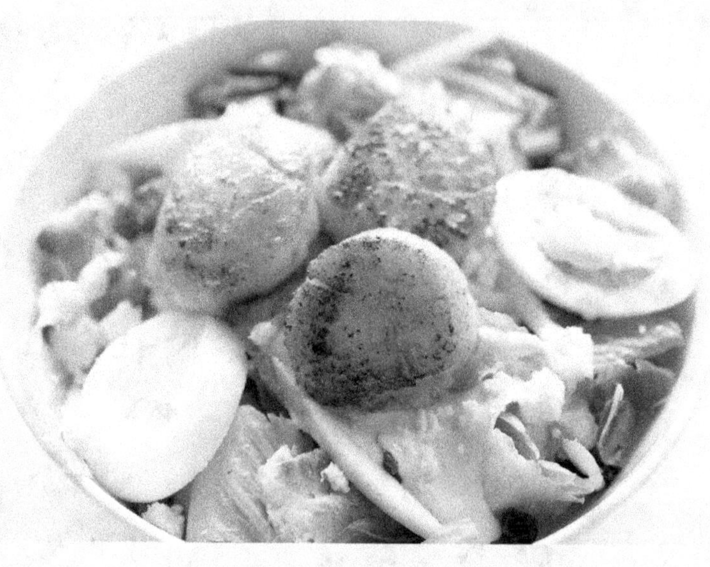

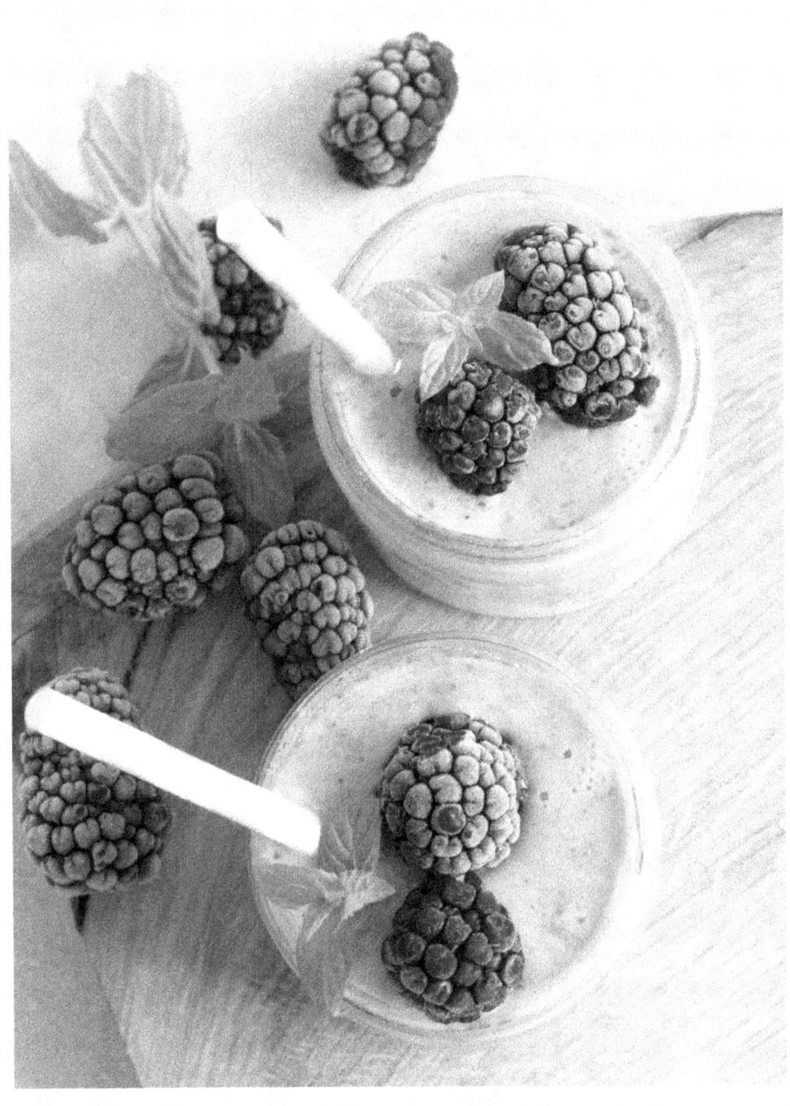

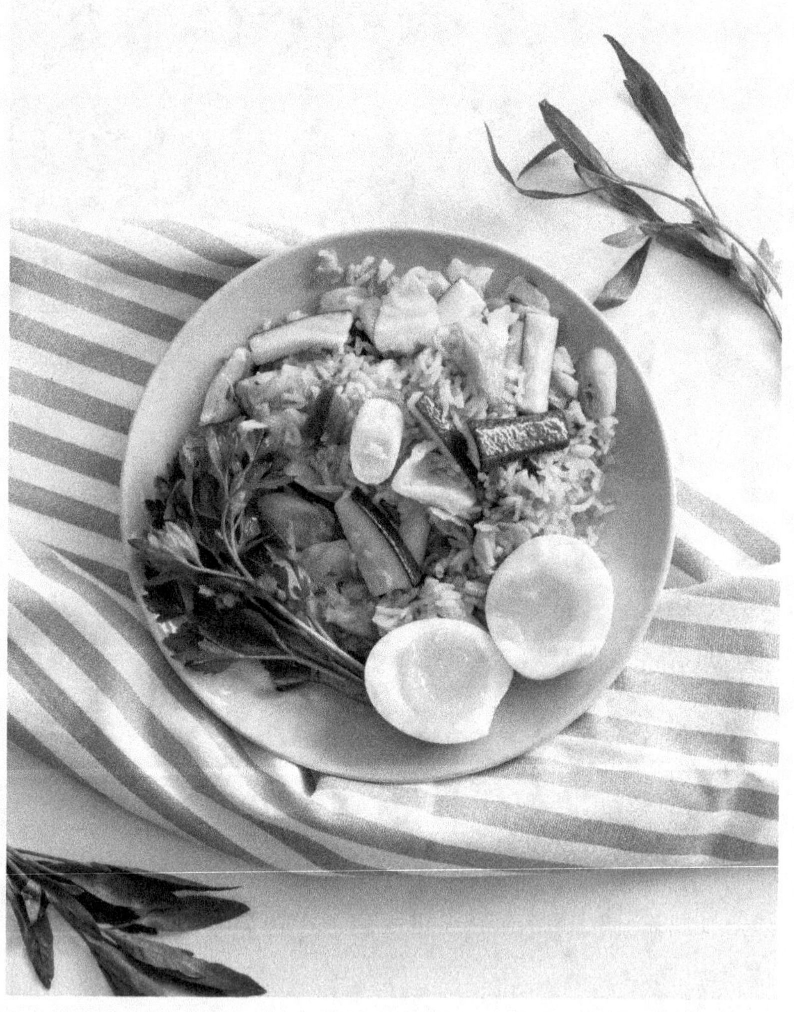

Author: Bright Liswaniso